This is Forty

THIS IS FORTY

LIVING AUTHENTICALLY

KORINA MAESTAS

Copyright © 2026 by Korina Maestas

All rights reserved.

No part of this book may be reproduced, distributed, or transmitted in any form or by any means, including photocopying, recording, or other electronic or mechanical methods, without the prior written permission of the publisher, except in the case of brief quotations embodied in critical reviews and certain other noncommercial uses permitted by copyright law.

This book is a work of nonfiction. The events, experiences, and reflections contained herein are shared from the author's perspective.

This book is not intended as a substitute for professional medical, psychological, or legal advice. Readers are encouraged to seek appropriate professional support when needed.

ISBN: 9798246397831

Printed in the United States of America

First edition

DEDICATION

This book is dedicated to the girl I once was—

the one who searched for love, safety, and belonging in all the wrong places,

and to the woman I became when I finally learned she was never broken.

To my husband, who taught me what safe love feels like—steady, patient, and real.

To my sister, who showed me what safety looks like simply by being there.

To my mother, who taught me that I am far stronger than I ever could have imagined.

And to my father—thank you for the ways you showed up, and for the lessons that shaped me.

To my children: you are the reason I chose healing.

You remind me that love can be gentle, consistent, and safe.

And to every woman who reaches forty feeling tired, unsure, or behind—

this is proof that it's not too late.

It's just the beginning.

AUTHOR'S NOTE

This book was written from the middle—not from arrival.

This is Forty is not a how-to, a redemption arc, or a declaration of having it all figured out. It is a reflection on what it means to stop surviving and start living with intention, honesty, and self-trust.

Some of the stories in these pages are personal. Others are emotional truths shaped by memory, time, and perspective. Names, identifying details, and timelines have been altered where necessary—not to change the truth, but to protect it.

This book does not offer neat conclusions. It offers permission. Permission to soften without failing. To question without unraveling. To rest without earning it. To choose yourself without apology.

If you are reading this at a moment of transition—between versions of yourself, between roles, between who you were and who you are becoming—know that you are not behind. You are exactly where growth happens.

Read slowly. Pause when you need to. Take what resonates and leave what doesn't. This book is not asking you to become someone new.

It is simply inviting you home.

ABOUT THE AUTHOR

Korina Maestas is a mother, author, and community builder devoted to helping women come home to themselves.

She is the founder and executive director of Kaibab Behavioral Services and Rising Mountain Academy, where she serves neurodivergent children, families, educators, and first responders through compassionate, evidence-based care. With a background in behavioral science and education, Korina's work bridges professional expertise with lived experience—always grounded in the belief that healing, belonging, and authenticity are not luxuries, but necessities.

Korina is also the author of On A Mother Level and This is Forty, books born from her own journey of survival, motherhood, leadership, and self-trust. Her writing speaks to women who are tired of performing strength and ready to live with honesty, softness, and intention.

After years of building organizations, raising children, and navigating chronic stress and personal healing, Korina's work has evolved into a larger mission: expanding the reach of compassionate care and reminding women that they are not broken—and never were.

She lives in Northern Arizona with her family, where she continues to write, lead, and advocate for a world where women are allowed to rest, to heal, and to take up space exactly as they are.

CONTENT NOTE

This book includes references to childhood trauma, substance abuse, emotional and physical abuse, self-harm, suicidal ideation, and loss. These experiences are discussed in a non-graphic, reflective manner in service of truth, healing, and understanding. Please take care of yourself as you read.

PROLOGUE

For most of my life, I believed survival was the goal.

Survive the chaos.

Survive the loneliness.

Survive versions of love that came with conditions, silence, or pain.

I spent my first forty years learning how to endure—how to read rooms before I read myself, how to earn belonging instead of trusting it was mine, how to shrink or perform or overgive in hopes that someone, somewhere, would finally stay.

I didn't know then that I was collecting lessons.

I only knew I was tired and feeling more pain than I could bear at times.

As I approached forty, something began to shift—not all at once, and not gently. It arrived through exhaustion. Through grief for the girl I once was. Through anger for the woman I had to become too fast. It came through motherhood, leadership, heartbreak, healing—and the quiet realization that I could no longer abandon myself to be loved.

Even now, I sometimes catch myself trying to earn the right to take up space.

Forty wasn't a breakdown.

It was a reckoning.

It was the moment I stopped asking What's wrong with me?

And started asking What's happening for me—and what do I choose now?

This is not a highlight reel.

It's a truth-telling.

It's about growing up wired differently in a world that rewarded compliance over compassion—where being "good," "easy," or "strong" often meant being invisible. It's about searching for love so desperately that harm masqueraded as connection. It's about abuse, silence, resilience, and the long road back to self-trust.

It's about motherhood, leadership, and the quiet weight women carry while still showing up for everyone else.

But most of all, this is a book about coming home to yourself.

This is Forty isn't about having it all figured out.

It's about choosing yourself with tenderness instead of punishment.

About self-acceptance replacing self-survival.

About realizing the lessons weren't wasted years—they were building blocks.

I am still unlearning.

Still choosing.

Still practicing compassion—especially toward myself.

If you feel behind…

If you're grieving the life you thought you'd have…

If you're rebuilding in the middle of adulthood…

You're not late.

You're exactly where you need to be.

This is the story of how I stopped living for approval and began living with intention—sometimes clumsily, sometimes bravely, but consciously, for the first time.

This is Forty.

And I'm not writing from the other side—

I'm writing from the threshold, inviting you to stand here with me.

1

TOO LOUD FOR QUIET ROOMS

Childhood — Sensitivity, Neurodivergence, and the First Lessons About Belonging

I remember the sound before I remember the feeling.

Pencils scratching across lined paper. The low hum of fluorescent lights vibrating just above my head. Chalk dust lingering in the air—sharp and powdery—clinging to my clothes long after the bell rang.

Most kids barely noticed any of it.

I noticed everything.

The world arrived at full volume. Every flicker, every sigh, every shift in tone registered in my body before my mind could catch up. I didn't have language for it then—no words like ADHD or sensory overload. I only knew my insides seemed calibrated differently.

Too alert.

Too responsive.

Too alive.

Too alone

I could feel tension in a room before anyone spoke. I sensed disappointment from across the hall. My energy moved faster than the expectations placed on me—legs bouncing, fingers tapping, thoughts spilling out before I could contain them.

Silence was required.

Stillness was rewarded.

And I struggled with both.

Adults called it "too much."

Calm down.

Pay attention.

Stop daydreaming.

So I learned to manage myself.

I sat on my hands so they wouldn't fidget. I bit my tongue when excitement rose too quickly. I practiced being smaller—quieter, more contained—learning early that shrinking myself made rooms feel safer.

At seven years old, I didn't know the word masking. I only knew belonging felt conditional.

When I laughed too loudly, I watched a teacher's eyes tighten and felt heat rush to my cheeks. When I did well on a spelling test, the praise felt fragile—earned, but temporary. Proof that I could belong, if only for the day.

Somewhere along the way, I learned to equate love with compliance.

Attention with performance.

Safety with self-control.

Home wasn't much quieter.

Rules were clear.

Emotions were not.

I learned to scan faces the way some children read storybooks—carefully, constantly—searching for clues about what was safe to say or feel. I moved through rooms on alert, attuned to shifts in mood and tone.

It felt normal then. Necessary.

Only later would I understand how exhausting that kind of vigilance becomes.

No one told me I was wired to feel deeply.

They told me I was dramatic.

So I buried my intuition beneath guilt and perfectionism. I learned to question my instincts, to override what my body knew in favor of what the world seemed to want from me.

Looking back now, I ache for that little girl. Looking back now, I see her.

She wasn't defiant or broken. She was responsive. She was trying to interpret a world that overwhelmed her senses and confused her heart.

She needed gentleness, not correction.

She needed someone to tell her that feeling deeply isn't a flaw—it's a form of intelligence.

There would be experiences later that complicated my relationship with my body and my voice—moments that reinforced the belief that I needed to manage myself to stay safe. But those come later.

What matters here is the beginning: the quiet shaping of a belief that followed me for decades—that who I was, unfiltered, was simply too much.

It would take years to unlearn the idea that belonging had to be earned, that my body and voice needed managing, that safety lived somewhere outside of me.

But this is where the story begins—not with healing, but with awareness. With the first knowing that I was never defective—only shaped by rooms that couldn't hold me yet.

When I meet children like her now—sensitive, restless, creative, radiant—I recognize the spark immediately. And I offer them what I once needed to hear:

You are not too much.

You are not a problem to be solved.

You are exactly enough for the world you're meant to build.

I will do everything I can to support you and create a safe place for you to thrive.

I wasn't too much. I was simply more than my environment knew how to hold.

2

THE PERFORMANCE OF BELONGING

What I Became to Survive

By the time I reached middle school, I understood something without ever being taught: belonging was not something you were given—it was something you earned.

Home had already taught me that love could be inconsistent, selective, and quietly withdrawn. Alcohol had a way of changing the rules without warning, and affection followed no predictable pattern. I learned early that needing too much felt dangerous—and that being myself did not guarantee safety.

So I adapted.

At school, I discovered a different system. Adults noticed me when I performed well—when I followed rules, when I achieved, when I succeeded. Praise arrived in neat handwriting, gold stars, and comments about how "mature" I was for my age.

Achievement brought stability.

Approval felt reliable there in a way it never did at home.

I became a high achiever not because I loved perfection—but because it worked.

Success became a language I could speak fluently. A way to be seen. A way to belong.

At home, love was not distributed evenly. My stepfather favored my sister—the quiet, obedient one. She took up less space, asked fewer questions, and didn't challenge shifting moods. In a house shaped by alcohol and emotional distance, her silence felt safer.

Watching her receive what I longed for taught me a painful lesson—or at least, that's how it felt in that house: love went to the child who needed less.

I was not that child.

I felt deeply. I reacted. I wanted reassurance. And so I turned that longing inward, believing something about me made love harder. The comparison didn't make me resent my sister—it made me turn against myself. I began to believe that if I could just become quieter, easier, more impressive, I might finally earn the care that always seemed just out of reach.

When achievement wasn't enough, I searched elsewhere.

I began seeking attention from boys—not recklessly, but earnestly. I wanted to feel chosen. Desired. Wanted for who I was, or at least for who I could become. I didn't yet have language for attachment or unmet longing. I only knew that being noticed, even briefly, softened the ache of feeling invisible.

At the same time, I struggled to find safety among my peers. I didn't fit easily with most of the girls at my school. The friendships I formed were often sharp-edged and conditional—cruelty disguised as closeness. Words were used strategically. Silence became punishment. Belonging always came with terms I never seemed able to meet.

By then, I wasn't just growing up.

I was performing.

I learned to read rooms quickly. To track moods. To adjust myself depending on who was watching. I became someone others might like because being myself had proven risky.

The mask wasn't about popularity.

It was about survival.

I learned that love could be earned through achievement.

That attention could be chased through desirability.

That safety depended on how well I managed myself.

What no one saw was the cost.

Every compliment felt temporary. Every success came with pressure to maintain it. Approval felt like something that could vanish the moment I disappointed, failed, or asked for too much. I learned to keep performing because stopping felt dangerous.

Belonging that depends on performance is fragile.

It disappears the moment you stop proving yourself.

I didn't know it then, but every role I played—successful student, agreeable presence, desirable girl—pulled me further from myself. Brick by brick, I built a wall that protected me from rejection while quietly isolating me from my own needs, feelings, and voice.

Looking back now, I see this with compassion: I wasn't performing because I wanted attention. I was performing because I needed connection. In a world where love felt conditional and approval felt safer than authenticity, I learned to become what was rewarded.

But survival strategies don't disappear just because the danger does.

They follow us—into relationships, careers, motherhood, leadership—until we pause long enough to ask the question that changes everything:

Who am I when I stop performing?

I learned to earn belonging—but I was worthy of it long before I proved anything.

3

THE EDGE OF ENOUGH

Teenage Years — Pain, Rebellion, and the Fight to Be Seen

By my teenage years, love had become something I needed to survive.

I couldn't be without a boyfriend. Being chosen by someone—anyone—felt like proof that I mattered. Alone, the emptiness was unbearable. And home made it worse.

Home wasn't a refuge.

It was a place where I learned how to brace myself.

There was no privacy.

No safety.

No place to rest.

Phone calls were listened to. Conversations weren't mine. Cameras watched my sister and me—not to protect us, but to monitor us. I learned early that silence didn't mean safety;

it meant scrutiny. I never knew when I was being watched, judged, or whispered about.

There was another home I imagined often—one where I felt accepted without condition. My father showed me a different kind of love. With him, I didn't feel like too much. I felt wanted. I longed to live with him, to be somewhere my nervous system could finally rest. But life didn't unfold that way, and wanting something didn't make it possible. So I carried that longing quietly, like a hope I didn't know how to ask for.

When I couldn't leave the house, I found safety where I could. Sometimes that safety was my sister. We learned how to protect each other in small, quiet ways—sharing rooms, sharing silence, sharing the unspoken understanding that we weren't imagining what was happening. Being near her made the house feel less dangerous, even when nothing else changed.

So I stayed gone as much as I could.

And when I walked back through that door, my body knew before my mind did.

Later, my mom told me he thought I was "unpredictable."

What I felt was rejection.

He told me he hated me.

Not once.

Not in anger that passed.

But repeatedly—like it was a truth he wanted me to carry.

When he drank, the air changed. His presence grew louder, heavier. I learned to read shifts in tone, to listen for footsteps, to calculate exits. There were nights he chased me through the house—my heart pounding, breath shallow, my body moving before my thoughts could catch up.

And the question that lived inside me—unanswered, relentless—was this:

Where was my mom?

Why didn't anyone stop it?

Why was I left to survive this alone?

I can see now that she was likely fighting her own battles with him—ones I didn't fully understand then. Survival can look like silence when you're trapped inside it. Knowing that doesn't erase the pain of what I needed and didn't receive, but it helps me hold the truth with more compassion than blame.

And beneath all of it lived another ache—the grief of knowing safety existed somewhere else, and not being able to reach it when I needed it most.

I didn't have language for what was happening to me.

I only had coping.

I used substances to escape the life I was living—to quiet the noise in my head, to numb the fear, to feel anything other than trapped. It wasn't rebellion the way people like to imagine it. It was desperation. A nervous system searching for relief.

When emotional pain became too heavy to carry, my body became the place it landed.

Self-harm wasn't about wanting to die.

It was about wanting the pain to move.

Emotional pain was everywhere—constant, invisible, suffocating. Physical pain was contained. Temporary. Something I could control. It gave my mind a single point of focus when everything else felt unbearable.

I wasn't seeking attention.

I was seeking quiet.

There came a moment—quiet enough it could have gone unnoticed—when I came dangerously close to not wanting to be alive anymore. Not because I wanted to die, but because I couldn't see how to keep living inside that much pain and no end in sight.

And then something unexpected happened.

I wanted to live.

Even then. Even there.

Not because life was good—but because I didn't want my story to end in that house. I didn't want my life defined by his hatred or by the silence that surrounded it. I wanted a future, even if I couldn't yet imagine what it looked like.

So I stayed.

I counted down the days like a prisoner marking time. Graduation wasn't a milestone—it was an escape plan. Every morning meant one day closer to leaving. One day closer to air.

But freedom didn't arrive gently.

Not long after graduation, I received flowers from my boyfriend—something kind, something simple. My stepfather was drunk again. I went searching the kitchen for a vase. He must have heard me, and his frustration escalated quickly, his voice sharp, his movements careless.

Then he drew a line straight through the house.

"There's your shit," he said, "and there's our shit."

In that moment, everything became clear.

I was never going to belong there.

I was never going to be safe there.

And staying would cost me more than I could afford to lose.

So I left.

Not healed.

Not whole.

But alive.

And for a girl who had been told she was unwanted, unpredictable, and unlovable—choosing to live was the bravest thing she had ever done.

When no one came to save me, I chose to save myself.

A LETTER TO THE GIRL STILL THERE

If you are reading this while still living in a house that hurts you, I need you to hear me.

> You are not crazy.
>
> You are not dramatic.
>
> You are not defective.

If you cling to love because it feels like oxygen, that doesn't make you weak—it means you are trying to survive without safety. If you numb yourself, escape, or find ways to quiet the pain, it doesn't make you bad. It means your nervous system is doing the best it can with what it has.

If you've learned to read faces before words, to listen for footsteps, to calculate exits—there is nothing wrong with you. You adapted to an environment that asked too much of you.

And if you've ever wondered whether it would be easier not to be here at all, know this:

Wanting the pain to stop is not the same as wanting to die.

There is a future beyond the walls you're living inside. There is a version of you who gets to choose peace, safety, and authenticity. You may not see her yet—but she is real, and she is waiting.

If there is even one safe adult you can tell, you deserve support.

If not, hold on however you can.

Staying alive is not weakness.

It is defiance.

One day, you will leave. And one day, you will look back and realize that surviving was the beginning of becoming.

You are not too much.

You were simply never protected enough.

And you are worth fighting for.

4

LOVE THAT HURT

The In-Between Years — When Longing Outpaced discernment

There is a season of life that exists between chapters—
after innocence, before clarity.
A place where desire speaks louder than instinct.
Where longing moves faster than discernment.

This was not a reckless time in my life.
It was a hungry one.

Somewhere between girlhood and womanhood, I learned how dangerous longing can be when it has gone unanswered for too long. When being seen feels rare, attention can masquerade as safety. When love has been inconsistent, intensity can feel like proof.

I didn't walk into these years unaware.
I walked into them hopeful.

I wanted to be chosen—not casually, not temporarily, but deliberately. I wanted to matter to someone the way I had spent my life trying to matter to others.

What I didn't yet understand was that my nervous system spoke a different language than my heart.
It wasn't searching for safety.
It was searching for familiarity.

Intensity felt like depth.
Certainty felt like protection.

I was drawn to men who felt consuming—magnetic, confident, sure of themselves. Their certainty steadied me. Their intensity made me feel alive. At the time, I believed that was passion. I believed closeness required surrender.

I had a way of drawing people in. I didn't know how to name it then—only that my openness, my depth, my eagerness to connect made people feel seen. Wanted. Chosen.

What I didn't yet understand was that attraction is not the same as safety.

This is where longing stopped feeling intoxicating—and started becoming expensive.

There was one relationship that came close to becoming permanent—close enough that marriage was discussed, planned for, imagined. From the outside, it looked like commitment. From the inside, I was steadily disappearing.

He didn't appreciate my body as it was. His desire came with conditions—preferences framed as opinions, expectations disguised as harmless commentary. I learned quietly that my body was something to be evaluated rather than accepted.

At the same time, trust was unraveling.

He cheated on me.
More than once.
And each time, he lied about it.

What hurt wasn't only the betrayal—it was the gaslighting that followed. The way the truth bent and shifted. The way my instincts were dismissed. The way I was encouraged to doubt what I felt in my body and replace it with his version of events.

When the truth surfaced, accountability didn't.

Instead, there were grand gestures. Expensive jewelry. Apologies wrapped in things instead of change. Attempts to repair without responsibility.

For a long time, I stayed. Not because I believed him—but because I believed love required endurance. I told myself that if I could just be understanding enough, flexible enough, forgiving enough, this could still work.

But something had already cracked.

I was losing myself trying to be chosen by someone who kept choosing elsewhere. My worth had become negotiable. My body, my trust, my voice—all of it conditional.

And then, for the first time, I did something different.

I left.

Not in anger.
Not in triumph.
But in clarity.

That decision didn't arrive loudly or confidently. It arrived quietly, carrying grief and fear and doubt—but also something new: self-respect. The beginning of self-trust.

I didn't yet have language for it, but I knew this much: love that requires you to disappear, to doubt your reality, or to accept repair without accountability is not love that can hold you.

This was not the relationship where I healed.
It was the relationship where I finally stopped abandoning myself.

I wanted love more than I understood safety.
That isn't weakness.
That is attachment shaped by absence.
That is trauma without a name.
That is a young woman doing the best she could with the tools she had.

I wasn't reckless.
I wasn't naïve.
I wasn't defective.

I was reaching—
for connection,
for protection,
for something steady enough to hold me.

Some lessons arrive gently.
Others leave bruises before they leave wisdom.

This was one of mine.

5

WHEN LOVE HURT MORE THAN LONELINESS

Early adulthood — the cost of staying

I didn't enter this season expecting harm.
I entered it believing I could handle whatever came.
By then, endurance felt familiar.
I had learned how to stay steady in uncertainty, how to adapt quickly, how to make myself smaller when needed. I mistook that skill for resilience. I believed that if something was difficult, it meant it mattered.

So when discomfort arrived, I normalized it.

I told myself this was what commitment looked like.
That love required patience.
That conflict was inevitable.
That discomfort was something mature people learned to tolerate.

What I didn't yet understand was how quietly self-abandonment can happen.

It didn't arrive all at once.
It arrived in small accommodations—choosing silence instead of honesty, flexibility instead of boundaries, understanding instead of self-respect.

I became skilled at minimizing my own reactions.
Explaining them away.
Talking myself out of what my body already knew.

I told myself stories to stay.

That this was normal.
That every relationship has edges.
That love requires work.

What I was really saying was: *I can handle this.*

And I could.

That was the danger.

Because being able to endure something doesn't mean it is safe.
It doesn't mean it is right.
It only means you have learned how to survive it.

My body knew long before my mind allowed it.
There was a constant vigilance—a quiet scanning, a readiness I couldn't turn off. My chest tightened before my thoughts caught up. My instincts whispered while my logic overruled them.

I learned how to override myself.

I confused survival with devotion.
Adaptation with loyalty.
Silence with strength.

From the outside, I appeared composed.
Capable.
In control.

From the inside, I was slowly disappearing.

There was no single moment that forced clarity.
No dramatic breaking point.

Just an accumulation of weight.

The realization that loneliness no longer scared me as much as staying did.
That the idea of being alone felt lighter than the cost of remaining unseen.

This chapter is not about blame—
not toward them, and not toward myself.

It is about context.

Because the truth is not that I ignored red flags.
The truth is that I had learned to live among them.

I wanted love more than I understood safety.

That isn't weakness.
That is attachment shaped by absence.
That is survival without a template for rest.

Eventually, something shifted.

Not loudly.
Not decisively.

But enough.

Enough discomfort.
Enough silence.
Enough negotiation.

I didn't yet know what healthy love looked like.
But I knew this wasn't it.

And for the first time, I allowed myself to imagine a life where staying wasn't the measure of my worth.

That awareness didn't save me overnight.
But it did something just as important.

It made leaving possible.

INTERLUDE

THE WEIGHT OF KNOWING

By the time I was twenty-five, I had already left the house. I had done what people often tell you to do when things are hard—get out, move on, create distance.

What no one tells you is that trauma doesn't always stay behind.

After I left, my stepfather's substance use didn't slow down. It escalated. What had once been unpredictable became dangerous. The chaos I had learned to navigate shifted onto my mother and sister, who were still living inside it.

This time, fear had teeth.

There were guns in the house.

There were threats that no longer sounded hypothetical.

There was a level of instability that tightened my chest even from far away.

I carried a quiet, unbearable knowing—the kind you don't say out loud because naming it feels like inviting it into existence. When he was arrested for drinking and driving, I didn't feel relief. I felt dread.

I knew it wasn't an ending.

It was a pause.

And I knew—deep in my bones—that when he was released, one of two things would happen:

Either someone else would die because of his drinking, or he would by his own choice.

There is no comfort in being right about something like that.

Not long after, he took his own life.

I won't describe the details, because they don't matter. What matters is the impact—the way the world felt quieter and heavier at the same time. His death didn't bring closure. It brought a complicated grief layered with fear, anger, sadness, and questions that never fully resolved.

What stays with me most is not just the loss, but the helplessness.

There is a particular kind of trauma in knowing something terrible is coming and being powerless to stop it. In watching danger unfold in slow motion. In understanding that love, addiction, and violence can coexist in the same person, and that none of it is something you can fix.

This wasn't the moment I fell apart.

It was the moment I learned how much I could hold.

I learned how to brace.

How to stay alert.

How to expect the worst and survive it anyway.

Those skills would later be praised as strength.

But at the time, they were simply survival.

And without realizing it, I carried them forward—into adulthood, into relationships, into places where love was supposed to feel safe.

There is a trauma in knowing—and still being unable to stop it.

6

WHEN SAFE LOVE WOKE ME UP

Early thirties — discovering safety and the cost of staying the same

Before my body demanded change, my life had already begun whispering it.

In my early thirties, I was recovering from a failed marriage. I began rediscovering who I was—turning inward in ways I never had before. Health and fitness became an obsession, and eventually, it led me to him. I experienced something I didn't know how to name at first—safe love. Not loud or intoxicating or consuming. Just steady. Kind. Predictable. Patient.

For the first time in my life, my nervous system wasn't bracing for impact.

I wasn't walking on eggshells.

I wasn't scanning for shifts in tone.

I wasn't wondering which version of myself I needed to be to stay connected.

And that safety did something unexpected—it revealed how unsafe love had felt before.

Trust didn't arrive all at once. It came in small moments and took years. Disagreements that didn't end in abandonment. Needs that were met without guilt. Silence that didn't feel dangerous. Each experience rewired something inside me, showing me that love didn't have to cost me myself.

Then, in my mid-thirties, I became a mother—and the awareness deepened.

Motherhood stripped away my ability to ignore patterns. I saw my own childhood through new eyes. I noticed how my body reacted before my thoughts could intervene. I recognized inherited survival responses surfacing in moments that should have felt simple.

There were times I caught myself responding from old wiring instead of present truth—and it terrified me.

Because suddenly, this wasn't just about me.

I looked at my child and understood something with painful clarity: I couldn't teach safety if I hadn't learned it myself. I couldn't model self-worth while still abandoning my own needs.

Love, I realized, is absorbed more than it is explained.

This is where the questions changed.

Not How do I keep pushing?

But Why do I believe I have to?

Not How do I manage it all?

But What am I showing my children about rest, worth, and belonging?

The awareness wasn't dramatic. It was quiet and persistent. A knowing that something in me needed to shift if the cycle was going to end here.

Safe love gave me the mirror.

Motherhood gave me the reason.

Together, they made one truth impossible to ignore:

Generational trauma doesn't break by accident.

It breaks by choice.

I didn't yet know how much my body would eventually demand that choice. I didn't know the cost of continuing to prove I was enough. But I knew—deep in my bones—that the old way could not be carried forward.

This is Forty is not about perfection or arrival.

It's about the moment healing becomes non-negotiable.

>The cycle ends with me.

7

BECOMING THE ONE WHO STAYS

Mid-thirties — choosing self-trust over self-abandonment

There comes a moment—quiet, almost imperceptible—when you realize you've spent much of your life leaving yourself.

Not in obvious ways.

Not in ways others could see.

But in the small, habitual ways that slowly teach a woman she must disappear to belong.

Leaving your body when it's tired.

Leaving your intuition when it speaks inconvenient truths.

Leaving your needs unspoken because they feel like a burden.

I learned early how to survive. Survival became my skill set—adaptability, vigilance, endurance. I learned how to read energy before words, how to anticipate moods, how to shape myself into what was needed in the moment. I learned that being agreeable felt safer than being honest, and that love was something you earned through effort, loyalty, and silence.

So I stayed busy.

I stayed capable.

I stayed useful.

What I didn't do was stay with myself.

From the outside, my life looked full—accomplished, impactful, strong. I was building, leading, advocating, holding space for others. I was praised for my resilience, admired for my grit.

And underneath it all lived a quiet exhaustion—one no amount of achievement could touch.

My body carried stories my voice had learned not to tell. There was a grief I couldn't yet name for the girl who learned too soon that her needs were negotiable.

Turning forty wasn't a collapse.

It was a reckoning.

Not with age—but with patterns.

I began to notice how often I left myself in moments that required honesty. How quickly I justified inconsistency. How deeply I confused endurance with love. How familiar chaos felt—and how peace sometimes made me restless.

I wasn't broken.

I was conditioned.

Conditioned to believe love was fragile.

Conditioned to believe worth was proven through sacrifice.

Conditioned to believe staying true to myself came at a cost.

Becoming the one who stays didn't happen dramatically. It happened slowly, through awareness. Through pauses. Through moments where my body asked for something different—and I finally listened.

I stopped asking, How do I keep going?

And started asking, What happens if I don't abandon myself here?

That question changed everything.

It changed how I worked—no longer worshipping burnout as devotion.

It changed how I loved—no longer mistaking intensity for intimacy.

It changed how I led—choosing integrity over image, alignment over approval.

And somewhere around this point—without a clear beginning or clean edges—my journey of forgiveness began.

Not forgiveness as a single act, but as a slow reorientation.

I didn't wake up ready to forgive. It emerged as I began to see my life through a wider lens. I started to understand that my trauma, while never deserved, had shaped the woman I became.

Not in spite of it.

Through it.

My experiences created the woman writing this book. They created the woman who notices what others overlook. The woman who advocates for those who feel unseen and unheard. The woman whose understanding of love is deep—not romanticized, but earned.

And eventually, they created the woman who learned how to forgive.

Forgiveness did not mean excusing harm or minimizing pain. It meant releasing the belief that my suffering was meaningless. It meant understanding that even the hardest experiences had expanded my capacity for compassion, leadership, and truth.

For the first time, I could hold my past without being consumed by it. I could grieve what I didn't receive while honoring what I became.

I began to see that everything in my life—even the moments that nearly broke me—had been shaping me.

Not happening to me.

But happening for me.

This realization didn't erase the past. It softened my grip on it. It allowed me to stay—fully, honestly, compassionately—with myself.

To stop outsourcing safety.

To stop asking others to give me what I had never learned to give myself.

Becoming the one who stays doesn't mean life becomes easy. It means you stop disappearing when things get hard. It means listening when your body whispers instead of waiting for it to scream.

It means choosing alignment over approval—even when that choice costs you roles, relationships, or identities that once felt essential.

Especially then.

At forty, I no longer measure love by how much I can tolerate.

I measure it by how safe I feel being fully seen.

I no longer confuse peace with passivity. I understand now that peace is built—through boundaries, through honesty, through self-trust.

And perhaps the most liberating truth of all:

I am not too much.

I was simply asking the wrong people to hold me.

Healing looks like this: I stay.

8

COMING HOME TO MYSELF

Motherhood — authenticity, regulation, and living from the inside out

For most of my life, I lived slightly outside of myself.

I learned how to adapt before I learned how to listen. How to perform before I learned how to rest. How to read a room before I ever asked what I needed. Survival taught me how to shape-shift, and for a long time, that skill kept me safe.

I didn't call it inauthenticity.

I called it strength.

Motherhood changed that—especially the kind of motherhood that does not follow the script.

Parenting a neurodivergent child stripped me bare in ways nothing else ever had. There was no performance that could carry me through the sleepless nights, the overstimulation, the advocacy, the constant calculations of safety, regulation, and love. No version of me could "hold it together" long enough to outrun the truth my body already knew.

This kind of motherhood demands presence, not perfection.

And presence requires honesty.

I remember the quiet moments—the ones no one sees. Sitting on the floor, exhausted, wondering if I was doing enough or doing it wrong. Grieving the ease I thought motherhood would have, while loving my child with a ferocity that terrified me.

Holding joy and heartbreak in the same breath.

There was guilt for wanting rest.

Fear for a future I couldn't predict.

Shame for struggling with something I loved so deeply.

And still—love.

Unconditional. Relentless. Grounding.

It was here that I could no longer abandon myself to keep things looking okay. My child didn't need a mother who performed strength or perfection. He needed a mother who was regulated, honest, and real.

And then there was my daughter.

She arrived two and a half years after her brother, carrying a different kind of medicine. Where my son asked me to heal so I could lead him safely through the world, my daughter offered me a love that felt instinctive, physical, undeniable.

She became my koala.

Always at my hip. Arms wrapped tight. Needing closeness not as reassurance, but as connection. She wanted my presence in a way that was embodied—my body, my attention, my steadiness. And in holding her, something in me softened that I didn't know was still guarded.

She loved me without performance.

Without expectation.

Without needing me to be anything other than here.

Her love didn't demand healing—it received it.

Even now, she is still my girl. Still needing me close. Still asking me to be present in ways that require slowing down, attuning, choosing connection again and again. And I love it—the invitation to stay, to practice presence instead of mastery.

My son showed me what had to change.

My daughter showed me what was possible.

Together, they anchored me in a truth my body could finally trust: that healing isn't only about breaking cycles—it's about learning how to receive love when it arrives without conditions.

That realization changed everything.

I began listening inward instead of outward. I stopped asking how I should show up and started asking how I could stay present. I learned that my authenticity—my groundedness, my softness, my boundaries—was not selfish.

It was necessary.

There is no prize for endurance.

No reward for suffering quietly.

No honor in disappearing.

There is only truth.

And truth is what allowed me to become the mother my child needed—and the woman I had always been trying to be.

Turning forty didn't make me fearless.

It made me honest.

Honest about my limits.

Honest about my needs.

Honest about the cost of pretending I was okay when I wasn't.

I stopped over-explaining.

I stopped apologizing for accommodations—mine or my child's.

I stopped performing resilience when what we needed was compassion.

And something steady took root.

The more I allowed myself to live authentically, the safer my child became—because children don't need perfect parents. They need regulated ones. Parents who trust themselves enough to slow down, advocate, and lead with truth instead of fear.

There was grief here.

Grief for the motherhood I imagined.

Grief for the years I spent trying to be everything to everyone.

Grief for how long it took me to realize that choosing myself was also choosing my child.

But there was relief too.

Because living authentically didn't take anything away from my motherhood.

It strengthened it.

This chapter of my life wasn't about becoming someone new.

It was about coming home—to my body, my truth, my values—so I could build a home where my children and I could all breathe.

This is what forty gave me:

A quieter strength.

A deeper trust.

A life lived from the inside out.

For the first time, I wasn't just surviving motherhood.

I was living it—fully, honestly, and in my own skin.

If you are parenting a child who needs more from you, you are not failing.

You are being invited to live more truthfully than you ever have before.

INTERLUDE

WHERE COMPASSION BECAME ACTION

For a long time, I believed gratitude and pain could not coexist.

Gratitude felt like betrayal—of the girl who suffered, of the woman who endured things she never should have had to survive. I worried that naming anything good that came from pain would somehow excuse it.

But gratitude, I've learned, does not mean approval. It means acknowledgment.

I do not feel thankful for what happened to me.
I feel thankful for what it taught me how to see.

I know what it is like to struggle quietly. To feel misunderstood. To live inside systems that reward compliance over compassion. To need support and not know how to ask for it—or worse, to ask and not receive it.

I know what it feels like to be overwhelmed by environments that were never designed with your nervous system in mind. To be labeled difficult instead of dysregulated. To be managed instead of understood.

That knowing never left me.

It followed me into adulthood. Into motherhood. Into rooms where children were being asked to adapt to systems that refused to adapt to them. Into conversations where behavior was addressed without curiosity, and compliance was mistaken for success.

And something in me recognized them.

The children who struggled.
The families who were exhausted.
The caregivers who felt unseen and unsupported.

I saw myself there—not in their diagnoses, but in their longing. Their need for someone to slow down, to listen, to advocate when their voices were dismissed or misunderstood.

I didn't choose this work because it was easy.
I chose it because it was familiar.

I knew what it felt like to need someone to stand between you and a world that asked too much. I knew how badly these children needed someone to say, You are not the problem. Someone willing to translate instead of punish. To protect instead of control.

Compassion became my language long before it became my profession.

Over time, that compassion took shape as action. As systems built differently. As spaces designed for regulation instead of restraint. As services rooted in dignity, safety, and trust. What began as understanding grew into responsibility.

This became my mission—not to save, but to serve.
Not to fix, but to advocate.
Not to manage behavior, but to expand care.

Expanding the reach of compassionate care is not just my professional work. It is personal. It is embodied. It is informed by every moment I wished someone had seen me sooner, understood me better, or stayed when it would have been easier to walk away.

Pain did not make me special.
But it did make me sensitive to suffering.

And that sensitivity—once framed as weakness—became the very thing that allowed me to do this work with integrity.

I do not believe everything happens for a reason.
But I do believe we get to decide what we carry forward.

I chose compassion.
I chose advocacy.
I chose to build what I once needed.

And in doing so, I found a way to hold my past without letting it define me—using it instead as a compass pointing toward care.

9

THE SOFTENING

Late thirties — releasing armor and redefining strength

For most of my life, strength meant survival.

It meant waking up and pushing through pain without naming it.

It meant adapting, achieving, producing—so no one would question my worth.

It meant staying busy enough that I never had to sit with what hurt.

Strength was armor.

And I learned early how to wear it well.

By the time I stood at the edge of forty, I had built what many would call a successful life. Businesses from the ground up. A career rooted in service and impact. Leadership roles that asked me to show up not only for myself, but for entire communities.

I became a mother who fought fiercely for her children.

A woman others looked to for answers, guidance, steadiness.

I was strong.

And I was exhausted.

Turning forty didn't arrive with fireworks or clarity wrapped in a bow. It didn't erase trauma or magically restore the parts of me worn thin by years of giving more than I had.

What it did—slowly, quietly—was something far more radical:

It gave me permission to soften.

For the first time, I stopped asking, How much more can I carry before I break?

And started asking, What am I allowed to put down and still be worthy?

This season of my life wasn't marked by achievement.

It was marked by honesty.

I began to notice how often I confused being needed with being loved. How easily I equated productivity with value. How deeply I believed rest had to be earned through exhaustion.

Forty asked me to unlearn that.

It taught me that self-acceptance doesn't arrive with applause. It arrives in the quiet decisions no one sees—choosing rest without justification, setting boundaries without apology, allowing myself to be human instead of heroic.

Compassion, I realized, isn't just a value I extend outward.

It is a practice I must turn inward.

I started releasing versions of myself that were born from survival—the overachiever, the fixer, the woman who never asked for help because she learned it wasn't safe to need.

I honored her for getting me here.

Then gently told her she could rest.

What remained was someone truer.

A woman who no longer needed to perform strength to be safe.

A woman who could say no and still feel whole.

A woman learning that softness is not the opposite of power—it is its refinement.

This season wasn't about healing everything.

It was about no longer abandoning myself in the process of living.

I learned that boundaries are not punishments; they are clarity.

That slowing down is not failure; it is discernment.

That my body's limits are not inconveniences—they are wisdom speaking.

"This is Forty" became less about age and more about arrival.

Arrival into self-trust.

Arrival into grace.

Arrival into a life where love, rest, and belonging were no longer things to be earned—but things I was finally willing to receive.

I am still ambitious.

I still dream boldly.

I still lead with fire.

But now I also lead with softness.

With intention.

With compassion for the woman I've been—and reverence for the one I am becoming.

And that—at last—feels like home.

10

THE BECOMING

Forty — living aligned, no longer negotiating belonging

By the time I reached forty, I wasn't searching for answers anymore.
I wasn't trying to understand my past, or make peace with it, or extract one last lesson from it.
I was learning how to live without carrying it everywhere I went.

There was a time when I believed growth always came with pain.
That if something wasn't hard, it wasn't meaningful.
That ease meant avoidance.
That peace meant I was missing something important.

Pain had been my teacher for so long that I didn't know who I was without its instruction.

Over time, I learned to appreciate what it gave me—depth, empathy, awareness, strength. I learned to forgive the people and seasons that shaped me. That mattered. It softened something inside me that had been clenched for decades.

But eventually, something quieter happened.

I stopped asking my pain to explain itself.

Not because it no longer mattered—
but because it no longer needed to.

I realized I had already learned what I was meant to learn.

For a long time, I thought honoring my past meant continually returning to it—extracting meaning, finding lessons, naming growth. I didn't understand that sometimes honoring your past simply means not living there anymore.

I didn't forget.
I didn't bypass.
I didn't rewrite the story.

I just stopped carrying it forward as proof.

Forty didn't arrive as a finish line.
It arrived as clarity.

Clarity that I am not broken.
Clarity that I was never defective.
Clarity that survival was never the goal—wholeness was.

There is a subtle difference between appreciating pain and allowing it to remain central. I can be grateful for the woman it shaped me into without letting it decide how I live now.

Forgiveness gave me release.
But this—this gave me agency.

I no longer need adversity to evolve.
I no longer need struggle to feel worthy of rest.
I no longer need intensity to feel alive.

I've learned to trust what feels steady.

There are mornings now when I notice my body before my to-do list.
I pause long enough to feel whether I'm tired or steady, rushed or grounded.
Sometimes the answer changes what I do next.

Some mornings, it means choosing twenty more minutes in bed—
snuggled in with my babies, furry and human—
letting presence matter more than productivity.

The difference is that I listen either way.

That alone feels like a kind of arrival.

These days, my life is quieter.
Not easier—just quieter.

I choose relationships that feel safe without fireworks.
I choose work that aligns instead of consumes.
I choose rest without narrating it.
I choose boundaries without over-explaining them.

There was a version of me who believed healing meant becoming someone new.

What I know now is that healing meant coming home—
and then building a life that didn't require me to leave
myself again.

I don't organize my life around what hurt me.
I don't lead with my wounds.
I don't measure my growth by how much I can endure.

I measure it by how present I am.

This is what forty looks like for me—not a triumphant
arrival, not a finished story, but a settled one.

A life where pain no longer has the loudest voice in the
room.
A life where forgiveness made space—but didn't demand
permanence.
A life where growth comes from attention, not suffering.

Nothing dramatic is happening now.

And that, finally, feels like enough.

EPILOGUE

This is not the end of my story.
It's the moment I stopped negotiating my place in it.

For a long time, survival looked like success.
If I could endure, adapt, keep moving, I believed I was doing life right.
I learned how to be strong before I learned how to be safe.
How to give before I learned how to receive.
How to become what was needed instead of who I was.

That way of living carried me far.
It also carried a cost.

There was a season when I thought healing meant understanding everything that had hurt me—naming it, forgiving it, finding the lesson so I could finally move on. And that work mattered. It loosened the grip of the past and softened what had been tight for years.

But I don't live there anymore.

At some point, I stopped asking my pain to keep teaching me.

Not because it failed—
but because its work was done.

I don't need my story to make sense to everyone.
I don't need my growth to be visible.
I don't need to keep proving that what I survived was real.

I am no longer organizing my life around what hurt me.
I am organizing it around what keeps me here.

Presence.
Rest.
Truth.
The quiet knowing of when enough is enough.

There are days when old patterns knock.
When fear resurfaces.
When my instinct is still to brace, to rush, to overfunction.

And now—
I notice.

I don't punish myself for it.
I don't turn it into a lesson.
I choose differently, and I move on.

This is what forty has given me.
Not certainty.
Not closure.

Choice.

The choice to stay with myself instead of disappearing.
The choice to listen instead of override.

The choice to let my life be ordinary and meaningful at the same time.

I am not waiting to become someone else.
I am not rehearsing my worth.
I am not surviving my life.

I am here.

And that is enough.

Made in the USA
Coppell, TX
25 February 2026

72742630R00062